THE Rapid 800

COOKBOOK

healthy way to lose weight fast

THE RAPID **800** COOKBOOK

Healthy Way To Lose Weight Fast

Copyright © Iota Publishing 2024

Images under licence from Shutterstock
All rights reserved. This book or any portion thereof may not be reproduced or used in any manner whatsoever without the express written permission of the publisher.

ISBN 978-1-913005-47-4

DISCLAIMER

Except for use in any review, the reproduction or utilisation of this work in whole or in part in any form by any electronic, mechanical or other means, now known or hereafter invented, including xerography, photocopying and recording, or in any information storage or retrieval system, is forbidden without the permission of the publisher.
This book is sold subject to the condition that it shall not, by way of trade or otherwise, be lent, resold, hired out or otherwise circulated without the prior consent of the publisher in any form of binding or cover other than that in which it is published and without a similar condition including this condition being imposed on the subsequent purchaser. The content of this book is available under other titles with other publishers.
This book is designed to provide information on a reduced calorie diet. Some recipes may contain nuts or traces of nuts. Those suffering from any allergies associated with nuts should avoid any recipes containing nuts or nut based oils. This information is provided and sold with the knowledge that the publisher and author do not offer any legal or other professional advice.
In the case of a need for any such expertise consult with the appropriate professional.
This book does not contain all information available on the subject, and other sources of recipes are available.
Every effort has been made to make this book as accurate as possible. However, there may be typographical and or content errors. Therefore, this book should serve only as a general guide and not as the ultimate source of subject information.
This book contains information that might be dated and is intended only to educate and entertain.
The author and publisher shall have no liability or responsibility to any person or entity regarding any loss or damage incurred, or alleged to have incurred, directly or indirectly, by the information contained in this book.

contents

Introduction — 5

Breakfast Dishes — 15
Banana & Strawberry Pancakes — 16
Bacon & Mushroom Pancakes — 17
Spanish Tortilla — 18
Oregano Peppers & Eggs — 19
Iced Mocha Frappuccino — 20
Wild Smoked Salmon, Avocado & Chives — 21
Banana & Coffee Smoothie — 22

Poultry Dishes — 23
Lemon & Tarragon Chicken — 24
Caribbean Chicken & Plantain — 25
Spanish Chicken Stew — 26
Almond & Walnut Chicken — 27
Indian Tikka Skewers — 28
Lean Turkey Burger — 29
Roast Garlic & Lemon Chicken Thighs — 30
Herbed Fried Chicken Livers — 31
Chicken & 'Noodles' — 32
Lime Chicken Fried 'Rice' — 33
Nutmeg & Cinnamon Chicken — 34
Spiced Spinach & Sunflower Seed Chicken — 35
Porcini Chicken & 'Rice' — 36
Chicken Drummers & Sweet Coleslaw — 37
South American Chicken Salad — 38

Beef, Lamb & Pork Dishes — 39
Chili Steak & Broccoli Stir-Fry — 40
Beef & Pineapple Salad — 41
Spicy Quarter Pounder — 42
Moroccan Lamb Casserole — 43
Italian Basil Meatballs — 44
Sausage & Chorizo Casserole — 45
Apple Pork & Coconut Garlic Mushrooms — 46
Sage Pork Fillet — 47

Minted Lamb & Carrots	48
Mini Indian Spiced Patties	49
Slow Cooked Oxtail Casserole	50
Red Thai Beef Curry	51
Bacon & Chili	52
Beef & Garlic Chaat	53
Sheik Kebab	54
Ground Lamb and Olives	55
Marinated Pork 'Medallions'	56

Seafood Dishes 57
Simple Coconut & Spinach Fish Curry	58
Avocado & Cilantro Fish Salsa	59
Pak Choi & Herb Scallops	60
Cajun Shrimp Salad	61
Seafood 'Noodle' Soup	62
Poached Wild Salmon & Tenderstem Broccoli	63
Pan Fried Asparagus & Tilapia	64
Spiced Prawns & Cauliflower 'Rice'	65
Japanese Tuna	66
Italian Bacon Mussels	67
Tandoori Shrimp Kebabs	68
Mediterranean Fish Stew	69
Stuffed Lemon Sole	70
Sweet Wild Salmon & Asparagus	71
Homemade Fish Goujons	72

Vegetable Dishes & Sides 73
Aromatic Cilantro Mushrooms	74
Basil & Vegetable Bake	75
Spiced Roasted Squash	76
Cauliflower 'Rice'	77
Zucchini 'Noodles'	77

High Intensity Interval Training (HIIT) Workouts & Stretches 79

nom nom
to eat something with great enjoyment.

If you want to make a change in your lifestyle that will improve your health and well-being, help you lose weight and reduce the risk of a range of degenerative diseases, then the RAPID 800 Diet could be for you. If you are also interested in the practice of fasting to kick-start weight loss or to maintain a healthy balanced weight long-term, then the RAPID 800 could be a perfect fit.

The RAPID approach to cooking requires a different mindset than the one you may have been used to so far, but don't be put off. It's really easy to pick up and this book will help you by keeping you on track with healthy ingredients every step of the way.

Traditionally, the RAPID 800 Diet does not focus solely on counting calories but instead on nutritious, balanced meals consisting mostly of lean proteins, vegetables, and healthy fats. However, taking these core dietary principles together with restrictive calorie counting by fasting for just two days a week, makes a powerful weight loss tool.
Let's begin by explaining the basic principles of the RAPID 800 Diet.

What Is the RAPID 800 Diet - in Simple Terms
The RAPID 800 Diet is an effort to return to a healthier way of eating that emphasizes whole foods and balanced nutrition. The diet consists mainly of lean proteins, vegetables, healthy fats, and some fruits and nuts. The modern diet, heavy in processed foods, refined sugars, and unhealthy fats, has led to various health issues including weight gain, food intolerances, and diseases like diabetes, heart disease, and more. The RAPID 800 Diet works with the biology of our bodies to make them work more efficiently. When our bodies work efficiently, they naturally burn fat. When they burn fat efficiently, they do not become overweight.

Why Avoid Certain Foods?
Refined sugars and processed foods (present in many modern convenience foods) are made up mainly of empty calories that provide little nutritional benefit. These foods can lead to spikes in blood sugar levels and are linked to weight gain and various health issues. Our bodies need carbohydrates to give us energy as they contain sugars, but these can also be found naturally in fruit and vegetables. The problem is when we consume too many processed carbs and sugars, the excess is stored as fat, leading to weight issues.

What Can I Eat on the RAPID 800 Diet?
Lots! Don't think of this as a restrictive diet!
- Lean Proteins - such as chicken, turkey, fish, and lean cuts of beef or pork.
- Fish - preferably wild-caught. Farmed fish can contain higher levels of mercury and toxins.
- Healthy Oils - such as olive oil and coconut oil.
- Fruit - in moderation, focusing on low-sugar options.
- Nuts - in moderation.
- Vegetables - especially leafy greens and non-starchy varieties.

What Should I Avoid?
- Refined sugars and processed foods (sweets, baked goods, sodas, etc.)
- Processed food.
- Alcohol in excess.

The good news is that we've already stripped the unhealthy ingredients from our recipes. All you have to do is follow the simple methods in our recipes to create some wonderful, appetizing, health-friendly meals.

Rapid 800
Fasting is probably most well-known as the 5:2 Diet - a great and flexible way to approach weight loss and less restrictive than many other diets. The 5:2 approach means you can eat 'normally' for 5 days a week and fast for 2. It's revolutionized the way people think about dieting.

By allowing you the freedom to eat normally for MOST of the week and fast by restricting your calorie intake for just TWO non-consecutive days a week (800 calories per day for men and women), you keep yourself motivated and remove that dreaded feeling of constantly denying yourself the food you really want to eat. It still takes willpower, but it's nowhere near as much of a grind when you know that you have tomorrow to look forward to. It's all about freedom. The ability to be flexible with the days you choose to fast makes the likelihood of you sticking to the diet for a prolonged period, or even indefinitely as a lifestyle choice, much higher than a regime that requires calorie restriction every single day.

Popularized by Dr. Michael J. Mosley, the 5:2 diet plan has been adopted as a way of life, which will change your relationship with dieting and weight loss. What's more, this way of eating is believed to have major health benefits, which could alter your health forever!

Initially, back in 2012 the 5:2 Diet was based on a 500 calorie limit on fast days. Since then further research and knowledge have grown into how fasting can help with weight loss and as such a newer approach of 800 calories on fast days is recommended – especially for those who may have already tried the 5:2 Diet but may have struggled to stick to 500 calories on their fast days. It may take a little longer to lose weight compared to the 500 calorie option but the positive aspect is that you are more likely to stick the plan long term.

It's important to remember what exactly a calorie is when controlling the number we consume.

- A calorie is a unit of energy.

Scientifically, 1 calorie is the amount of energy required to raise one gram of water by one degree Celsius. To you and me, a calorie (a unit of energy) is a vital component of our body and its health. We need energy to go about our every day tasks and for our body to function and repair itself as it should. So energy (calories) are a necessity and are present in everything we eat – carbohydrates, protein and fat. We know that excess calories are linked to weight gain and poor health so maintaining a healthy level of calories or reducing calories to accelerate weight loss should be managed carefully and safely.

The main difference between the original 500 calorie option and the new 800 rule (apart from the additional 300 cals) is the period of actual fasting. On the 800 plan you should include a 14 hour fast period either directly after your fast day or directly before you fast day.
So for example if you choose Monday as a fast day you might have an evening meal on Sunday at 6pm then completely fast until breakfast on Monday morning at 8am.

Alternatively fast for your 14 hour period following your last meal on your fast day. E.g. dinner at 5pm on Monday with breakfast on Tuesday at 7am.
Flexibility is the great thing about the 5:2 Diet but remember your fast days should be on 2 non-consecutive days and you must fast for a 14 hourperiod either before or after.

On your non-fast days, you can eat 'normally' without counting calories but try to follow a healthy diet – you can still choose any of the recipes in this book on your non-fast days – just don't worry about counting the calories. You should enjoy your non-fast days but don't binge! Avoid processed food, snacking between meals and the usual temptations like fizzy drinks, biscuits, crisps, chocolate and alcohol.

How It Works
The concept of fasting is an ancient one and modern science is uncovering evidence that fasting can be an extremely healthy way to shed extra weight. Research has shown that it can reduce levels of IGF-1 (insulin-like growth factor 1, which leads to accelerated ageing), activate DNA repair genes, and reduce blood pressure, cholesterol and glucose levels as well as suggestions of a lower risk of heart disease and cancers.

Fasting works by restricting your body to fewer calories than it uses. Most importantly is that it does this in a way that remains healthy and is balanced by eating normally for the other 5 days of the week.

This book has been developed specifically to help you prepare your fast day RAPID 800 meals, however, if you want to find out more about the specific details behind the science of 5:2 Diet fasting we would recommend studying Dr. Michael J. Mosley's work and, as with all diets, you should consider seeking advice from a health professional before starting.

If you are pregnant, breastfeeding, diabetic, suffer from any eating disorder, or are under the age of 18 we do not recommend this diet for you. If you suffer from any health issues you should first seek the advice of a health professional before embarking on any form of diet.

The RAPID 800 Diet

Now that you understand the basic principles of healthy living and the RAPID 800, the journey to a healthier and slimmer lifestyle is simpler.

This book will give you a wide choice of delicious, single-serving, calorie-counted, healthy meals that will not only form the basis of your 800 calorie fast plan but will also open your eyes to a new lifestyle choice that will help you lose weight and in the long term, improve your overall health and immune system.

This book has been designed to provide a wide selection of easy-to-prepare recipes to keep you motivated and your engine stoked during your fasting day and, because you can eat normally for the 5 days a week, you'll be much more likely to stick with it over time and enjoy the long-term health and weight benefits.

Simply choose your fast day meals from any of the tasty recipes using the calories for each dish. You can choose any combination as long as your don't exceed 800 calories through the day (remember any drinks you consume throughout the day will count towards your 800 cals and don't forget the 14 hour fast period).

When Can I Expect To See Results?

By the end of your first week in most cases! Obviously everybody is different, but where someone is carrying extra weight they will normally see a reduction in the first week of embarking on fasting. Typically many will see greater weight loss at the beginning, followed by a slowing down, then eventually settling around a stable healthy weight. For optimal results, we recommend following the RAPID 800 plan for at least 6 weeks so you can begin to appreciate the health benefits and see noticeable weight loss results.

Taking It Week By Week

The 5:2 Diet can work for you whatever your lifestyle. Each week you should think carefully about which days are likely to be best suited to your fasting days and then stick with it (remembering to factor in your 14-hour fast period). You can change your fast days each week or keep a regular routine, whichever suits you best. Ideally, your fasting days should be non-consecutive. This gives you the opportunity to stay motivated by eating normally the following day, although it can be acceptable to fast for 2 days consecutively if you are feeling particularly inspired.

Give yourself the best possible chance of success by choosing your fast days in advance and sticking to them. As we have already said, we recommend choosing two non-consecutive fasting days so that you only have one 24-hour period at a time where you have to concentrate on limiting your calories.

Of course, reducing your calorie intake for two days will take some getting used to and inevitably there will be hunger pangs to start with but you'll be amazed at how quickly your body adapts to your new style of eating.

How Will I Manage My Calorie Intake?

There are two different approaches to managing your 800 calorie intake on your fast days depending on your personal preferences and lifestyle.

- OPTION 1: Skip breakfast, eat lunch & dinner.
- OPTION 2: Skip lunch, eat breakfast and dinner.

There is much research and debate about the health benefits and risks of skipping meals, however the beauty of the 5:2 Diet is that the fasting occurs only for 2 days of the week with the remaining 5 reserved for 'normal' eating and recommended daily calorie intakes (1900-2000 for women, 2400-2500 for men). This means there is not a prolonged period of starving the body of calories, and eating balanced meals like those included in this book ensures that nutrition is still provided on the fasting days.

You may choose meals from any chapter as long as they stay under 800 calories. Remember that drinks during the day such as tea and coffee will also count towards your calorie limit so remember to account for these. You can also make some meals more substantial if you need to increase calories by adding side dishes (see the suggestions at the end of this introduction).

Portion Sizes
The size of the portion that you put on your plate will significantly affect your weight loss efforts. Filling your plate with over-sized portions will obviously increase your calorie intake and hamper your dieting efforts.

It's important that with all meals, both on your fasting and normal eating days, you use a correct sized portion, which generally is the size of your clenched fist. This applies to any side dishes of vegetables and carbs too. You will be surprised at how quickly you will adopt this as the 'norm' as the weeks go by and you will begin to stop over-eating.

Some Fasting Tips
- Avoid too much exercise on your fasting days. Eating less is likely to make you feel a little weaker, so don't put the pressure on yourself to exercise.
- Don't give up! Even if you find your fasting days tough to start with, stick with it. Remember you can eat 'normally' tomorrow.
- Drink plenty of water throughout the day. Water is the best friend you have on your fasting days. It's good for you, has zero calories, and will fill you up and help stop you feeling hungry.

- When you are eating each meal, put your fork down between bites – it will make you eat more slowly and you'll feel fuller on less food.
- Drink a glass of water before and also with your meal. Again this will help you feel fuller.
- Brush your teeth immediately after your meal to discourage yourself from eating more.
- Have clear motivations. Think about what you are trying to achieve and stick with it. Remember you can eat what you want tomorrow.
- If unwanted food cravings do strike, acknowledge them, then distract yourself. Go out for a walk, phone a friend, play with the kids, or paint your nails.
- Whenever hunger hits, try waiting 15 minutes and ride out the cravings. You'll find they pass and you can move on with your day.
- Remember - feeling hungry is not a bad thing. We are all so used to acting on the smallest hunger pangs that we forget what it's like to feel genuinely hungry. Feeling hungry for a couple of days a week is not going to harm you. Learn to 'own' your hunger and take control.
- If you feel you can't do it by yourself then get some support. Encourage a friend or partner to join you on the 5:2 Diet. Having someone to talk things through with can be a real help.
- Get moving. Being active isn't a necessity for fasting to have results but as with all diets increased activity will complement your weight loss efforts. Think about what you are doing each day: choose the stairs instead of the lift, walk to the shops instead of driving. Making small changes will not only help you burn calories but will make you feel healthier and more in control of your weight loss.
- Don't beat yourself up! If you have a bad day forget about it, don't feel guilty. Recognise where you went wrong and move on. Tomorrow is a new day and you can start all over again. Fast for just two days a week and you'll see results. Guaranteed!

Calorie Conscious Side Suggestions

If you want to make any of the recipes or snacks in this book more substantial you may want to add an accompaniment to them. Over the page is a list of some key side vegetables, salad etc which you may find useful when working out your calories.

All calories are per 100g/3½ oz. Rice & noodle measurements are cooked weights.

Considerations

It's worth bearing in mind that you may have to adjust cooking times. Meat and vegetables are rarely uniform in size and appliances in each household can differ, so a slight alteration in cooking times may be required. Just monitor the cooking process and use your own judgment.

As we pointed out earlier in the book, all the recipes adhere to the broad modern approach to healthy living. You will no doubt find many discussions as to exactly what does and does not constitute a healthy diet. What is helpful to remember is that you need to follow a diet that works for you. All of the recipes in this book are health-friendly. Feel free to replace any ingredients to your own taste or based on your own approach to a healthy lifestyle.

Exercise Plan

If you are interested in complementing your new healthy eating lifestyle with a workout plan you'll find a manageble collection of High Intensity Interval Training workouts at the back of the book. This is a super fast and really effective way to exercise. Short, intense bursts of exercise with rests in between make your heart work harder, increases cardio strength, improves metabolism and as a result helps your body burn more calories both during and after your workout.

Initially we recommend doing the workouts only on your non-fast days. As you progress through the 6 week plans you can exercise on any day you choose.

- Asparagus: 20 cals
- Brussel Sprouts: 42 cals
- Butternut Squash: 45 cals
- Cabbage: 30 cals
- Carrots: 41 cals
- Cauliflower: 25 cals
- Celery: 14 cals
- Courgette/zucchini: 16 cals
- Cucumber: 15 cals
- Leeks: 61 cals
- Mixed salad leaves: 17 cals
- Mushrooms: 22 cals
- Pak choi; 13 cals
- Parsnips: 67 cals
- Pepper (bell): 20 cals
- Rocket: 17 cals
- Spinach: 23 cals
- Sweet corn: 86 cals
- Tomatoes: 18 cals

The Rapid 800

breakfast
dishes

Banana & Strawberry Pancakes

SERVES 1

- 1 tsp butter
- 1 large egg
- 1 ripe banana
- 1½ tbsp peanut butter
- 4 ripe strawberries

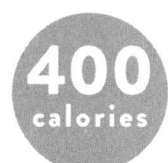

- Use a fork to mash up the peeled banana and combine well with the peanut butter. Beat the egg into the mixture until you have a smooth texture.

- Heat the butter in a frying pan and, when hot, put the mixture in the pan in two mounds, which will spread out to make two small, thick pancakes. Cook for 2 mins each side or until cooked through.

- Slice the strawberries and serve over the top of the warm pancakes.

You could use the mixture to make a single, larger pancake is you prefer.

Bacon & Mushroom Pancakes

SERVES 1

- 2 tsp olive oil
- 1 large egg
- 2 slices lean back bacon
- 50g/2oz mushrooms, sliced
- 1½ tbsp almond butter
- 1 tbsp freshly chopped flat leaf parsley

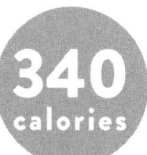

340 calories

- Combine the egg well with the almond butter until you have a smooth texture.

- Heat half the oil in a frying pan and cook the bacon & mushrooms until golden. Keep the bacon and mushrooms warm while you make the pancakes.

- Add the rest of the oil to the pan and heat well. Put the mixture in two mounds which will spread out to make two small thick pancakes. Cook for 2 mins each side or until cooked through.

- Serve the bacon and mushrooms on top of the pancake and sprinkle with chopped parsley.

You could use the mixture to make a single larger pancake is you prefer.

Spanish Tortilla

SERVES 1

- 2 tsp olive oil
- 2 onions
- 3 slices chorizo

- 1 garlic clove
- 2 large eggs
- Sea salt & pepper to taste

325 calories

- In a food processor whizz together the chorizo, onion and garlic. Use a small frying pan to gently sauté the onion mixture in a little olive oil for 5-10 minutes until softened.

- Beat the eggs in a bowl, pour the onions and chorizo from the pan into the bowl with the eggs, season and combine well.

- Add a little more oil to the frying pan and pour the egg mixture into the frying pan. Cover and leave to cook on a very low heat for 4-5 minutes until golden underneath.

- Carefully flip the omelette and cook for a further 4-5 minutes until the omelette is firm to the touch.

Use a small frying pan for this recipe to make a thick omelette/tortilla, which you can cut into wedges for eating hot or cold.

Oregano Peppers & Eggs

SERVES 1

- 2 tsp olive oil
- 3 large eggs
- ½ red pepper, sliced
- ½ red onion, chopped
- 2 tbsp freshly chopped oregano
- Sea salt & pepper to taste

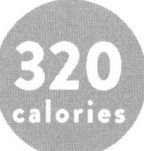

320 calories

- Heat the oil in a frying pan and gently sauté the peppers and chopped onions for a few minutes until softened.

- Meanwhile beat the eggs and oregano together along with some seasoning. Pour into the pan and stir continually until the eggs set.

- Serve immediately.

Any sweet peppers are fine in this recipe; you could also use baby shallots rather than red onion for a sweeter taste.

Iced Mocha Frappuccino

SERVES 1

- 1 cold shot espresso
- 120ml/ ½ cup milk
- Handful ice cubes
- 1 tbsp cocoa powder

75 calories

- Add all the ingredients to a blender and whizz to the desired consistency.
- Pour into a tall glass and add more ice if required.

This is a lovely refreshing morning drink that you can prepare ahead and store in the fridge.

Wild Smoked Salmon, Avocado & Chives

SERVES 1

- 50g/2oz wild smoked salmon slices
- ¼ cucumber, cubed
- ½ ripe avocado, sliced
- ½ red onion, thinly sliced
- 3 radishes, finely sliced
- 2 tbsp freshly chopped chives
- 1 tbsp lemon juice
- 1 tbsp olive oil
- Sea salt & pepper, to taste

325 calories

- Arrange the fish and salad together on the plate.
- Sprinkle the lemon juice on the salmon and season with pepper.
- Sprinkle the avocado oil over the salad and top with the chives.
- Serve immediately.

Smoked salmon, lemon juice and freshly ground black pepper are an unbeatable classic combination.

Banana & Coffee Smoothie

SERVES 1

- 1 cold shot espresso
- Handful ice cubes
- 2 tbsp cocoa powder
- 120ml/½ cup milk
- ½ tsp vanilla extract
- 1 tsp runny honey

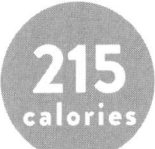

215 calories

- Add all the ingredients to a blender and whizz to the desired consistency.
- Pour into a tall glass and add more ice if required.

Smoothies are a great start to the day. This recipe should be sweet enough but you can add a little more honey if you want to.

The Rapid 800

poultry
dishes

Lemon & Tarragon Chicken

SERVES 1

- 1 tbsp olive oil
- 150g/5oz skinless, chicken breast
- 1 garlic clove, crushed
- 2 tsp freshly chopped tarragon
- 1 lemon
- Pinch crushed chilli flakes
- 75g/3oz rocket leaves
- Sea salt & pepper to taste

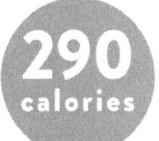

290 calories

- Chop half the lemon into slices, squeeze and reserve the juice from the other half. Combine the lemon juice, olive oil, garlic, tarragon and chilli flakes together to create a marinade.

- Place the chicken breast in an ovenproof dish and score the flesh with a knife. Brush the breast with all the marinade, season well and leave covered in the refrigerator for up to 1 hour.

- Preheat the oven to 200C/400F/Gas Mark 6.

- Carefully cover the chicken breast with the sliced lemon pieces. Place in the oven and cook for 30-40 minutes or until the chicken is cooked through.

- Remove the cooked chicken to a plate and serve with the rocket salad.

If there is any marinade left in the bowl after cooking, spoon it onto the salad as a dressing. This dish is also good with chopped fresh tomatoes tossed through the rocket leaves.

Caribbean Chicken & Plantain

SERVES 1

- 1 tbsp olive oil
- 1 onion, chopped
- 125g/4oz skinless, chicken breast
- 75g/3oz plantain, peeled & sliced
- 1 tsp almond flour
- 1 garlic clove, crushed
- 1 tsp freshly grated ginger
- ½ tsp each cayenne pepper, paprika & mustard seeds
- Pinch ground cinnamon
- 60ml/¼ cup chicken stock
- 120ml/½ cup coconut milk
- 1 portion cauliflower rice (p77)
- Sea salt & pepper to taste

450 calories

- Preheat the oven to 180C/350F/Gas Mark 5.
- Gently sauté the onion, garlic, dried spices and mustard seeds in the olive oil for a few minutes until the onion softens and the mustard seeds begin to pop.
- Stir the almond flour through the onions, add the hot chicken stock and continue stirring for a minute or two.
- Combine all the ingredients, except the coconut milk in an ovenproof dish. Place in the oven and leave to cook for 40-45 minutes or until the chicken is cooked through and the plantain is tender.
- Stir through the coconut milk, season and serve with the cauliflower rice.

Plantain is a starchy type of banana, which must be cooked before eating and is used widely in Caribbean cooking. They are readily available in the US & UK.

Spanish Chicken Stew

SERVES 1

- 2 tsp olive oil
- 125g/4oz skinless, chicken breast, sliced
- 1 onion, chopped
- 1 tsp each smoked paprika & dried sage
- 1 tsp each freshly chopped rosemary & basil
- 200g/7oz chopped tomatoes
- 1 yellow pepper, sliced
- 75g/3oz uncooked chorizo sausage, sliced
- 2 garlic cloves, crushed
- 8 pitted olives, halved
- 50g/2oz tenderstem broccoli, roughly chopped
- Sea salt & pepper to taste

510 calories

- Preheat the oven to 200C/400F/Gas Mark 6.

- Gently sauté the onion, sliced pepper, garlic, sage & paprika in the olive oil for a few minutes until softened. Add the sliced chorizo & chicken and cook for 3-4 minutes longer.

- Combine all the ingredients in an ovenproof dish. Place in the oven and leave to cook for 30-40 minutes or until the chicken is cooked through and the vegetables are tender.

- Season well and serve.

As an alternative you could try shredding the chicken after cooking and serve warm or cold on slices of bread.

Almond & Walnut Chicken

SERVES 1

- 1 tbsp olive oil
- 150g/5oz skinless chicken breast
- 1 tsp ground almonds
- 1 tbsp walnuts, finely chopped
- 50g/2oz mushrooms, chopped
- ½ onion, finely chopped
- 1 tsp garlic paste
- Sea salt & pepper to taste

330 calories

- Preheat the oven to 200C/400F/Gas Mark 6.

- First mix together the ground almonds, olive oil, walnuts, mushrooms, onion & garlic paste.

- Make a lengthways slit in the chicken breast and stuff with the walnut mixture. Don't worry if it's overflowing just gently cover in foil to keep it together.

- Place in an ovenproof dish and leave to cook for 35-40 minutes or until the chicken is cooked through. Season well and serve.

A crispy crunchy onion salad served on the side is a lovely addition to this meal.

Indian Tikka Skewers

SERVES 1

- 150g/5oz skinless, chicken breast, cubed
- 1 tbsp yoghurt
- 1 tsp each ground cumin, turmeric, coriander & chilli powder
- 1 garlic clove, crushed
- 2 metal skewers
- 1 romaine lettuce, shredded
- ½ red onion, sliced
- ½ lemon cut into wedges
- Sea salt & pepper to taste

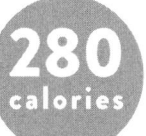
280 calories

- Season the cubed chicken. Mix together the spices, garlic & yoghurt. Add the chicken, combine well, cover and leave to chill for an hour or two in the refrigerator.
- Skewer the chicken pieces to make 2 chicken kebabs and place under a medium/high grill for 6-8 minutes each side, or until the chicken is cooked through (take care handling the skewers as they will get hot).
- Serve with the shredded lettuce, sliced red onion and lemon wedges.

If you don't have time to leave the chicken to marinate don't let that put you off making this dish. It will still taste good.

Lean Turkey Burger

SERVES 1

- 1 tsp olive oil
- 125g/4oz lean, turkey mince
- 1 egg yolk
- ½ onion
- 1 garlic clove
- 1 tbsp freshly chopped parsley
- 1 handful shredded lettuce
- 1 ripe tomato, sliced
- 1 burger bun
- Sea salt & pepper to taste

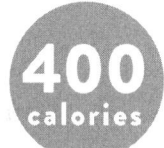

400 calories

- Place the garlic, onion, turkey mince, egg and parsley in a food processor. Pulse for a few seconds until combined. Season well and form into a large burger patty about 2cm/1inch thick.

- Brush with the olive oil and place under a medium/high grill for 6-8 mins each side, or until the burger is cooked through.

- Split the burger bun and serve with tomato and lettuce on top.

It's worth investing in a plastic burger maker to make perfect burgers shapes. They cost very little and really improve the shape and texture of the patty.

Roast Garlic & Lemon Chicken Thighs

SERVES 1

- 1 tsp olive oil
- 250g/9oz skinless chicken thighs
- 150g/5oz sweet potatoes, cubed
- ½ parsnip, cubed
- ½ carrot, cubed
- ½ onion chopped
- 2 vine ripened tomatoes, halved
- 2 garlic cloves, crushed
- 2 tbsp lemon juice
- 2 tsp runny honey
- Sea salt & pepper to taste

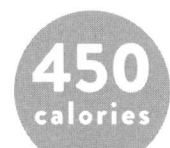
450 calories

- Preheat the oven to 200C/400F/Gas Mark 6.

- Mix together the olive oil, garlic, lemon juice and honey. Brush the chicken thighs and tomatoes with the honey mixture and use the rest to coat the vegetables well in an ovenproof dish.

- Season, place everything in the oven, except the tomatoes, and leave to cook for 30-40 minutes or until the chicken is cooked through and the vegetables are tender.

- Halfway through cooking add the tomatoes.

- Season well and serve.

You could add a garnish of freshly chopped rosemary to this lovely dish.

Herbed Fried Chicken Livers

SERVES 1

- 1 tbsp olive oil
- 1 tbsp butter
- 200g/7oz chicken livers
- 100g/3½oz, mushrooms sliced
- 1 onion, chopped
- 1 tbsp balsamic vinegar
- 2 garlic cloves, crushed
- 1 tbsp each freshly chopped thyme & rosemary
- Sea salt & pepper to taste

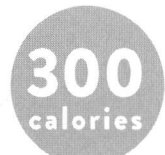

- First slice the chicken livers lengthways and remove the hard connective tissues from the center. Season and lay out on a plate.

- Meanwhile gently sauté the garlic, onions and mushrooms in the oil and butter for a few minutes. Increase the heat and add to the pan along with the chopped herbs and balsamic vinegar. Cook for 4-6 minutes or until the livers are cooked through but not tough.

- Season and serve.

Take care not to burn the herbs. You could cook the livers in a separate pan from all the other ingredients and combine at the end if preferred.

Chicken & 'Noodles'

SERVES 1

- 1 tbsp olive oil
- 150g/5oz skinless chicken breast
- 4 tbsp flour
- 1 tsp each ground garlic, onion powder, cumin & paprika
- ½ tsp cayenne pepper
- 1 large egg
- 1 large zucchini/courgette
- Sea salt & pepper to taste

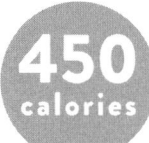

- Prepare the zucchini noodles (see page 77).
- Combine together the flour and dried spices in a shallow bowl.
- Beat the egg and pour onto a plate.
- Roll the chicken breast in the flour and egg repeatedly in turn to build up a layered coating. Finish with the flour as the outer coating.
- Heat the oil in a pan and fry the chicken breast for 6-8 minutes each side.
- Add the noodles to the pan for the last 2-3 minutes and fry until the chicken is cooked through and the noodles are tender.

The flour and egg batter should give you a nice crisp coating to the chicken.

Lime Chicken Fried 'Rice'

SERVES 1

- 1 tbsp olive oil
- 150g/5oz chicken breast, cubed
- 1 red onion, chopped
- ½ tsp each turmeric, cumin & paprika
- ½ red chilli, finely chopped
- 2 tbsp lime juice
- 2 tbsp freshly chopped cilantro (coriander)
- ½ head cauliflower

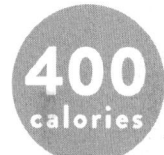

400 calories

- Prepare the cauliflower rice (see page 77).
- Gently sauté the onions, chilli, cumin, turmeric & paprika in a frying pan with the olive oil.
- Add the chicken, 'rice', lime juice & chopped cilantro and cook for 6-10 minutes or until the chicken is cooked through.
- Season and serve.

Cauliflower 'rice' is a really useful addition to the Rapid 800 diet.

Nutmeg & Cinnamon Chicken

SERVES 1

- 1 tsp olive oil
- 150g/5oz skinless chicken breast
- ½ tsp each ground garlic, paprika, cinnamon & nutmeg
- 3 shallots, sliced
- 125g/4oz tenderstem broccoli
- ½ cup chicken stock
- Sea salt & pepper to taste

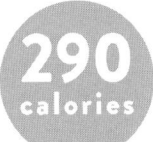

290 calories

- Preheat the oven to 200C/400F/Gas Mark 6.
- Mix together the dried spices and rub them all over the chicken breast.
- Brush the broccoli and spiced chicken with the olive oil. Season well and put in an ovenproof dish. Pour in the stock, cover and place in the oven.
- Leave to cook for 40-50 minutes or until the chicken is cooked through and the broccoli is tender.

Having the chicken covered keeps the steam circulating around the meat and makes it tender.

Spiced Spinach & Sunflower Seed Chicken

SERVES 1

- 1 tsp olive oil
- 125g/4oz chicken breasts
- ½ tsp dried crushed chilli flakes
- 1 tsp each ground cumin, garlic powder, paprika & basil
- 125g/4oz spinach leaves
- 2 tbsp sunflower seeds
- 1 avocado, sliced
- 2 tbsp lemon juice
- Sea salt & pepper to taste

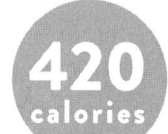

420 calories

- Toast the sunflower seeds in a dry pan until browned.

- Mix together half the olive oil, all the ground paprika, garlic powder, cumin & basil and rub into the chicken. Put the chicken under a medium/hot grill and leave to cook for 10-15 minutes or until cooked through.

- Meanwhile heat the rest of the oil in a saucepan. Add the spinach, seasoning and the chilli flakes. Cook for 2-3 minutes, stirring throughout, until the spinach wilts.

- Arrange the cooked chicken, spinach and sliced avocado on a plate, sprinkle the lemon juice and sunflower seeds over the top and serve.

Also try chicken thighs which are a darker meat prized as one of the tastiest parts of the bird.

Porcini Chicken & 'Rice'

SERVES 1

- 1 tbsp olive oil
- 125g/4oz chicken breast, cubed
- 2 slices lean, back bacon, sliced
- ½ onion, chopped
- 2 garlic cloves, crushed
- 1 tbsp balsamic vinegar
- 60ml/¼ cup chicken stock
- 3 tbsp dried porcini mushrooms
- ½ head cauliflower
- 2 tbsp freshly chopped flat leaf parsley
- Sea salt & pepper to taste

360 calories

- First place the porcini mushrooms in a little warm water and leave for 10-15 minutes to rehydrate (reserve the mushroom water and use to make the stock).
- In a food processor whizz the cauliflower until it is the size of rice grains.
- Use a frying pan to cook the chopped bacon and chicken in the olive oil for 5 mins.
- Add the onion, stock, vinegar, porcini mushrooms and garlic to the pan; stir and season well.
- Cook for 5 minutes and add the cauliflower 'rice'.
- Cook until the liquid is reduced, the chicken cooked through and the cauliflower tender. Season and serve sprinkled with flat leaf parsley.

You could add some chopped sundried tomatoes to this dish and cook along with the bacon for an alternative flavor.

Chicken Drummers & Sweet Coleslaw

SERVES 1

- 2 tsp olive oil
- 2 chicken drumsticks
- 2 tsp runny honey
- 1 tsp each garlic powder, Chinese five spice & paprika
- ½ white pointed/Chinese cabbage
- 2 carrots, peeled and grated
- 1 red onion
- 1 red chilli, deseeded
- 2 tbsp lime
- 1 tbsp fish sauce
- 1 tsp maple syrup
- 1 tbsp olive oil
- 2 tbsp freshly chopped coriander

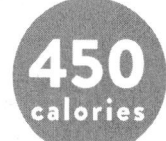

- Mix together the honey, olive oil, garlic powder, paprika & Chinese five spice and brush over the chicken. Place the drumsticks under a medium/high grill and cook for 10-15 minutes or until cooked through.

- Meanwhile shred/chop the cabbage, red onion and carrots to make a coleslaw texture (you could pulse in a food processor if you are short of time).

- Mix together the lime juice, chilli, olive oil, fish sauce and syrup into a dressing. Stir the dressing through the shredded vegetables, sprinkle with chopped coriander and serve on the side with the cooked chicken drumsticks.

Feel free to alter the balance of fish sauce, lime and syrup in the dressing to suit your own taste.

South American Chicken Salad

SERVES 1

- 150g/5oz cooked chicken
- 2 stalks celery, chopped
- ½ red onion, sliced
- 1 tbsp avocado oil
- 1 tbsp water
- 2 garlic cloves
- 1 small egg
- 2 tsp runny honey
- 1 tsp each lemon juice, cumin, sea salt & paprika
- 2 red chillies, deseeded
- 1 romaine lettuce, shredded
- Sea salt and pepper, to taste

- First shred the cooked chicken with two forks and mix with the celery and raw red onion slices in a bowl.

- Place all the other ingredients, except the romaine lettuce, in a blender and whizz until you have a smooth dressing.

- Stir the dressing through the chicken and onions. Pile on top of the romaine lettuce and serve.

The dressing for this salad is inspired by chipotle ready-made sauce.

The Rapid 800

beef, lamb & pork dishes

Chilli Steak & Broccoli Stir-Fry

SERVES 1

- 1 tbsp olive oil
- 150g/5oz lean sirloin steak
- 1 garlic clove, crushed
- ½ tsp each ground ginger and crushed chilli flakes
- 1 red chilli, deseeded and finely chopped
- 2 spring onion/scallions, sliced
- 150g/5oz tenderstem broccoli, roughly chopped
- 100g/3½oz ready prepared stir-fry vegetables
- Salt & pepper to taste

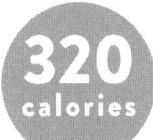
320 calories

- Season the steak and slice into small strips. Stir-fry in the olive oil for 60 seconds on a high heat.
- Add the rest of the ingredients and continue to stir-fry for 2-3 minutes until the steak is cooked to your liking.

Stir frying for just a few minutes will keep the broccoli crunchy and the steak tender. Try reducing or increasing cooking time to suit your own taste.

Beef & Pineapple Salad

SERVES 1

- 1 tbsp olive oil
- 150g/5oz beef fillet steak
- 1 tsp brown sugar
- 2 slices pineapple, finely chopped
- 1 carrot, cut into matchsticks
- 1 tbsp freshly chopped mint
- 1 tbsp fish sauce
- 1 tbsp rice wine vinegar
- 1 red chilli, deseeded and finely chopped
- 2 garlic cloves, crushed
- 100g/3½oz rocket

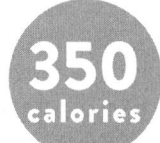

- Mix together one clove of garlic, the sugar & olive oil and brush onto the steak.
- Mix together the other garlic clove, fish sauce, chopped chilli, chilli flakes and pineapple to make a dressing.
- Meanwhile fry the steak on a high heat in a dry pan for 2 minutes each side (more if you prefer well-done).
- Remove from the pan and rest while you combine the salad.
- Toss the pineapple dressing, rocket and carrots together.
- Thinly slice the steak and place on top of the rocket mix.
- Sprinkle with chopped mint and serve.

This dish is best when the steak is cooked medium-rare, however you can alter to suit your taste.

Spicy Quarter Pounder

SERVES 1

- 1 tsp olive oil
- 125g/4oz lean ground/mince beef
- 1 egg
- ½ onion
- 1 garlic clove
- ½ tsp each ground cumin, turmeric and paprika
- 1 tsp mustard
- 1 ripe tomato, sliced
- 1 handful shredded lettuce
- 1 burger bun
- 1 tsp mustard
- Sea salt & pepper to taste

400 calories

- Place the garlic and onion in a food processor and pulse. Add the mince, spices & egg and pulse for a few seconds until combined.

- Season well and form into a large burger patty. Brush with olive oil and place under the grill on a medium/high heat for 5-7 minutes each side or until the burger is cooked through.

- Meanwhile gently toast the bun and spread on the mustard.

- Serve with tomato and lettuce on top.

Try cayenne pepper rather than paprika for an extra 'kick'. Plastic burger moulds make perfect burger shapes, improving the shape & texture of the patty.

Moroccan Lamb Casserole

SERVES 1

- 1 tbsp olive oil
- 150g/5oz lean lamb fillet, cubed
- ½ onion, chopped
- 1 carrot, cut into thin matchsticks
- 1 tsp each ground cumin & coriander
- ½ tsp each ground cinnamon & chilli powder
- 1 red pepper, sliced
- 1 garlic clove, crushed
- 50g/2oz dried apricots, chopped
- 200g/7oz tinned chopped tomatoes
- 1 tbsp tomato puree/paste
- 1 tbsp flat leaf parsley, chopped
- Sea salt & pepper to taste

450 calories

- Preheat the oven to 180C/350F/Gas Mark 5.

- Gently sauté the onion, peppers, carrots, garlic & spices in the olive oil for a few minutes until softened. Add the chopped tomatoes & cubed lamb and cook for 3-4 minutes longer.

- Combine all the ingredients, except the chopped parsley, in an ovenproof dish. Place in the oven, cover and leave to cook for 50-60 minutes or until the lamb is tender and cooked through.

- Season well and serve with the chopped parsley sprinkled over the top.

The spices in this Moroccan inspired dish will fill your kitchen with delicious warming smells.

Italian Basil Meatballs

SERVES 1

- 1 tbsp olive oil
- 150g/5oz lean ground/mince beef
- 1 egg
- ½ onion
- 1 garlic clove
- ½ tsp each ground cumin, turmeric and paprika

- 1 tsp dried oregano
- 2 tbsp freshly chopped basil
- 250ml/1 cup tomato passatta/sieved tomatoes
- ½ tsp each sea salt & brown sugar
- Sea salt & pepper to taste

- Preheat the oven to 200C/400F/Gas Mark 6.

- Place the garlic and onion in a food processor and pulse. Add the mince, spices, herbs & egg and pulse until well combined. Season and form into small meatballs with your hands.

- Place in an ovenproof dish and cook for 10-15 minutes.

- Meanwhile combine together the passatta, salt & sugar. Add to the meatballs, mix well and continue to cook for a further 10-15 minutes until the meatballs are cooked through and the sauce is piping hot.

Meatballs are a staple of Italian food which have become a firm family favorite in the US & UK. Serve with a salad or 'rice' (click here for 'rice' recipe)

Sausage & Chorizo Casserole

SERVES 1

- 1 tbsp olive oil
- 1 lean pork sausages, sliced
- 1 uncooked chorizo sausages, sliced
- ½ onion, chopped
- 1 red pepper, sliced
- 125g/4oz cauliflower florets
- 1 tsp each mixed dried herbs & paprika
- 200g/7oz tinned, chopped tomatoes
- 2 garlic cloves, crushed
- 2 tbsp tomato puree/paste
- Salt & pepper to taste

460 calories

- Preheat the oven to 200C/400F/Gas Mark 6.
- Gently sauté the onion, sliced pepper, garlic & herbs in the olive oil for a few minutes until softened. Add the sausages & chorizo and cook for 3-4 minutes longer.
- Combine all the ingredients in an ovenproof dish and cook for 30-40 minutes or until the sausages are cooked through and the cauliflower is tender.
- Season well and serve.

Chorizo sausage comes as either a cooked 'salami' type sausage or as an uncooked sausage which must be cooked before eating. Use the uncooked variety for this dish.

Apple Pork & Coconut Garlic Mushrooms

SERVES 1

- 1 tbsp olive oil
- 150g/5oz pork loin steak
- 2 tbsp cider vinegar
- 1 eating apple, peeled & chopped
- 2 garlic cloves, crushed
- 100g/3½oz mushrooms, sliced
- 2 tbsp coconut cream
- 75g/3oz shredded vegetable ribbons
- Sea salt & pepper to taste

390 calories

- Season the pork loin steak and brush with a little olive oil. Place in an ovenproof dish under the grill at a medium/high heat and grill for 3-4 mins each side.

- Meanwhile gently sauté the chopped apple, garlic and mushrooms in the olive oil for a few minutes until softened. Stir through the vinegar & coconut cream and pour over the pork steak (use the same pan for the vegetables later). Reduce the heat under the grill and cook for a further 4-6 minutes or until the pork is cooked through.

- Meanwhile use the same sauté pan to gently cook the vegetable ribbons for a few minutes in any leftover juices from the mushroom mixture.

- Serve the cooked loin with the vegetables on the side.

Pan-ready shredded vegetables are widely available and really useful to have in the refrigerator.

Sage Pork Fillet

SERVES 1

- 2 tsp olive oil
- 150g/5oz piece pork tenderloin
- 60ml/¼ cup chicken stock
- 1 orange, juiced
- 1 garlic clove, crushed
- 1 tbsp freshly chopped sage
- 125g/4oz butternut squash, peeled & cut into small cubes
- 50g/2oz spinach, chopped
- Sea salt & pepper to taste

340 calories

- Preheat the oven to 180C/350F/Gas Mark 5.

- Season the pork tenderloin, brush with olive oil and quickly brown all over in a frying pan for a few minutes.

- Place in an ovenproof dish with all the other ingredients and cover tightly. Cook for 30-35 minutes or until the pork is cooked through and the squash is tender.

- Remove the pork and cut into thick slices. Arrange on the plate with the spinach and squash to the side.

- Pour the stock and orange juices over the top of the pork and vegetables and serve.

Some vegetables can take longer to cook than meat. Ensure the squash is cut into small enough pieces so that it is tender once the pork is cooked.

Minted Lamb & Carrots

SERVES 1

- 1 tbsp olive oil
- 150g/5oz lean lamb fillet, cubed
- 2 tbsp balsamic vinegar
- ½ tsp each garam masala, ground turmeric, coriander
- 1 garlic clove, crushed
- 3 carrots, chopped
- 1 red onion, sliced
- 2 tbsp freshly chopped mint
- 60ml/¼ cup lamb stock
- Sea salt & pepper to taste

380 calories

- Preheat the oven to 200C/400F/Gas Mark 6.

- Season the lamb and quickly brown all over in a frying pan with the olive oil for a few minutes. Place in an ovenproof dish with all the other ingredients and cover tightly.

- Cook for 40-45 minutes or until the lamb is cooked through and the carrots are tender.

This is lovely served with flat breads to mop-up the delicious cooking juices.

Mini Indian Spiced Patties

SERVES 1

- 1 tbsp olive oil
- 150g/5oz lean lamb mince
- ½ tsp each ground coriander, garlic, salt, paprika, cumin & turmeric
- ½ onion, very finely chopped
- 1 green chilli, very finely chopped
- 1 tbsp freshly chopped mint
- 2 tsp lemon juice
- 1 pitta bread
- 1 romaine lettuce
- 2 vine ripened tomatoes, finely chopped
- Sea salt & pepper to taste

320 calories

- Gently sauté the onion, green chillies, coriander, paprika, cumin, turmeric and garlic in the olive oil for a few minutes.

- Place the mince, lemon juice, chopped mint and warm spicy onion mixture into a food processor and whizz together. Take the mixture out, divide into 5-6 portions and shape into small flat meat patties. Brush with a little olive oil and place under the grill on a medium/high heat for 4-5 minutes each side or until the lamb is properly cooked through.

- Serve inside the pitta bread with the lettuce and tomatoes.

This dish is known as Shami Tikka in traditional Indian cooking.

Slow Cooked Oxtail Casserole

SERVES 1

- 1 tbsp olive oil
- 250g/9oz beef oxtails
- ½ onion, chopped
- 1 carrot, chopped
- 75g/3oz mushrooms
- 1 garlic clove, crushed
- 1 tsp each freshly grated ginger & ground all spice
- ½ tsp each dried crushed chilli flakes
- 250ml/1 cup beef stock, homemade
- 60ml/¼ cup cream
- 3 tbsp freshly chopped flat leaf parsley
- Sea salt and pepper

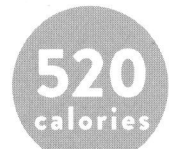

- Gently sauté the onions, carrots, garlic and ginger in a frying pan with the oil for a few minutes until softened.

- Add all the ingredients, except the cream & parsley, to an ovenproof dish. Cover tightly and leave to cook for 3-4 hours or or until the oxtail is tender and falls off the bone (ensure it does not dry out by adding more stock if needed).

- When cooked stir through the cream, sprinkle with parsley and serve.

Oxtail has a rich, deep taste which is really brought out by slow cooking.

Red Thai Beef Curry

SERVES 1

- 1 tbsp olive oil
- 150g/5oz sirloin steak, thinly sliced
- 1 garlic clove, crushed
- ½ onion, chopped
- 1 tbsp Thai red curry paste
- 1 carrot, cut into thin matchsticks
- 3 tbsp freshly chopped coriander
- 120ml/½ cup coconut milk
- 1 tsp fish sauce
- 1 portion cauliflower rice (see page 77)
- Sea salt & pepper to taste

390 calories

- Gently sauté the onions, carrots and garlic in the olive oil for a few minutes until softened.

- Increase the heat, add the curry paste and stir-fry the steak for 2 minutes with all the other ingredients, except the chopped coriander. Simmer gently for 10-12 minutes or until everything is cooked through and tender.

- Serve with cauliflower rice and sprinkle with fresh coriander.

Simmer the coconut milk gently to ensure it does not 'split' and spoil the dish.

Bacon & Chilli

SERVES 1

- 1 tbsp olive oil
- 150g/5oz lean, minced ground beef
- ½ onion, finely chopped
- 2 garlic cloves, crushed
- 1 tsp each paprika, onion powder & chilli powder
- 200g/7oz tinned chopped tomatoes
- 250ml/1 cup beef stock
- 75g/3oz sweet potatoes, peeled & finely chopped
- 1 tsp lime juice
- 2 tbsp tomato puree/paste
- 2 slices back bacon, finely sliced
- 1 large egg
- Sea salt & pepper to taste

480 calories

- Brown the mince for a few minutes in some of the olive oil. Remove to a plate and gently sauté the onion and garlic for a few minutes.

- Add the mince back to the pan along with the dried spices, chopped tomatoes, beef stock, sweet potatoes and tomato paste. Simmer well for 10-20 minutes or until the beef is cooked through, the vegetables tender and the stock has reduced to a thick sauce.

- Meanwhile in a separate pan cook the bacon in the rest of the olive oil until crisp and brown. 1 minute before serving break the egg into the bacon pan on a high heat. Stir through the bacon to make a scrambled egg and bacon mix.

- Plate up the beef and serve the egg and bacon mix on top.

You could also add some freshly chopped parsley or chives to this dish to serve.

Beef & Garlic Chaat

SERVES 1

- 2 tbsp olive oil
- 200g/7oz sirloin beef, cubed
- ½ tsp sea salt
- 4 cloves garlic, crushed
- 1 tsp ground coriander, turmeric and mild chilli powder
- 2 tbsp lemon juice
- 2 tbsp freshly chopped coriander
- 1 crisp lettuce, shredded
- 1 red onion, cut into rings
- Sea salt & pepper to taste

380 calories

- Add the olive oil to a pan and stir fry the beef pieces for 2-3 minutes.
- Add the salt, garlic, coriander, turmeric & chilli powder. Cook for a minute longer or until the beef is cooked to your liking.
- Remove from the heat and stir in the lemon juice.
- Serve with the green and red onion salad.

Chaat is the term to describe savory food which is typically served as street-food in Pakistan and India. This simple beef dish is delicious fast-food.

Sheik Kebab

SERVES 1

- 1 tbsp olive oil
- 150g/5oz lean ground lamb mince
- ½ tsp ground coriander, garlic, salt
- ½ onion, very finely chopped
- 1 green chilli, finely chopped
- 1 tbsp freshly chopped mint
- 1 tbsp lemon juice
- 4 wooden skewers

320 calories

- Leave 4 wooden skewers to soak in water for a few hours.
- Gently sauté together the onion, green chillies, coriander and garlic in the olive oil for a few minutes.
- Place the lamb, lemon juice, chopped mint & warm spicy onions in a food processor. Whizz together until well mixed. Take the mixture out and place on a chopping board.
- Divide into 4 portions and roll into long sausage shapes around each skewer.
- Grill under a medium heat for 12-15 minutes or until the lamb is properly cooked through.

Lean mincemeat and light spices make this a lovely super-quick dish, best served with a plain salad.

Ground Lamb & Olives

SERVES 1

- 1 tsp olive oil
- 150g/5oz ground lamb mince
- 3 shallots, chopped
- 1 garlic clove, crushed
- 1 tsp each dried basil, oregano, paprika & garlic powder
- ½ tsp ground allspice
- 1 zucchini/courgette, chopped
- 10 black pitted olives, halved
- 3 fresh tomatoes, finely chopped
- 1 tbsp tomato puree/paste
- 60ml/¼ cup lamb stock
- ½ tsp dried crushed chilli flakes
- Sea salt & pepper to taste

360 calories

- Sauté the lamb, garlic, shallots & ground spices in the olive oil for a few minutes.
- Add all the other ingredients to the pan, cover and simmer for 20-30 minutes or until the lamb is cooked through and the sauce is thick.

It's fine to use mild onions if you don't have shallots. Also tinned tomatoes will work well rather than fresh.

Marinated Pork 'Medallions'

SERVES 1

- 1 tbsp olive oil
- 175g/6oz pork tenderloin medallions
- 1 tbsp each freshly chopped rosemary & thyme
- ½ tsp each sea salt and paprika
- 4 garlic cloves, crushed
- 1 lemon, cut in two
- 100g/3½oz kale
- Sea salt & pepper to taste

320 calories

- Combine together the olive oil, chopped herbs, salt, paprika, garlic & lemon juice (from one of the lemon halves). Brush the mix liberally over the pork medallions. Cover and leave to marinate for a few hours or overnight.

- When ready to cook place the meat and marinade juices in a dry frying pan on a medium high heat and cook on each side for 3 minutes or until cooked through.

- Meanwhile steam the kale for 8-10 minutes or until tender. Squeeze the other lemon half and mix the juice with the kale and plenty of sea salt & pepper.

Pork Medallions are thick slices of meat from the pork tenderloin.

The Rapid 800

seafood dishes

Simple Coconut & Spinach Fish Curry

SERVES 1

- 150g/5oz skinless, boneless, fresh cod fillet
- 125g/4oz spinach leaves
- 1 tbsp olive oil
- 2 garlic cloves, crushed
- 200g/7oz tinned chopped tomatoes
- 60ml/¼ cup coconut cream

- ½ red onion, chopped
- 1 green chilli, deseeded and finely sliced
- ½ tsp each sea salt, ground ginger, garam masala, paprika, turmeric, chilli powder & cumin

380 calories

- First cut the fish fillet into strips and sprinkle with the sea salt.

- Gently heat the oil in a pan and fry the onion, spices & garlic for a few minutes.

- Add the fish and chopped tomatoes and cook for 5-7 minutes or until the fish is cooked through.

- Stir in the spinach leaves & coconut milk and warm through for a few minutes until the spinach is wilted.

Take care when heating the coconut cream as you do not want it to 'split' and spoil.

Avocado & Cilantro Fish Salsa

SERVES 1

- 150g/5oz skinless, boneless, fresh cod fillet
- 2 tsp olive oil
- ½ cucumber, peeled & finely diced
- 1 avocado, peeled & diced
- 2 vine ripened tomatoes, finely diced
- 1 fresh lime, squeezed
- 3 tbsp freshly chopped cilantro (coriander)
- 1 onion, finely chopped
- 1 red chilli, deseeded & finely chopped
- ½ tsp each sea salt & black pepper
- 75g/3oz rocket leaves

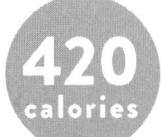

420 calories

- Combine together the cucumber, avocado, tomatoes, lime juice, onion, chilli, coriander and sea salt to make a fresh salsa dressing.

- Season the cod fillet with black pepper. Heat the olive oil in a frying pan and gently cook for 5-6 minutes or until the fish is cooked through.

- Remove to a plate and serve with the salsa piled on top and the rocket leaves on the side.

Cod is listed as the ingredient in this recipe but any type of firm meaty white fish fillet will do well in this dish.

Pak Choi & Herb Scallops

SERVES 1

- 5 large fresh scallops
- 50g/2oz pancetta/Italian bacon, cubed
- 1 tsp each freshly chopped oregano & thyme
- 1 tsp paprika
- 2 garlic cloves, crushed
- ½ lemon, cut into wedges
- 1 pak choi, cut in half lengthways
- ½ tsp crushed chilli flakes
- 1 tbsp olive oil
- Sea salt & black pepper to taste

310 calories

- Combine the scallops together with the oregano, thyme & paprika.

- Heat the olive oil in a frying pan and add the bacon, garlic, chilli flakes and pak choi. Cook for aprox 5-7 minutes until the bacon begins to crisp and the pak choi halves are browned and tender. Remove to a dish and keep warm for a few minutes whilst you cook the scallops.

- Use the same frying pan to gently fry the scallops for 6-10 minutes until they are cooked through, add a little more oil if needed.

- Remove to a plate and serve with the lemon wedges, pak choi and bacon on the side.

Pak choi is a wonderful Asian vegetable widely available in the UK & US. If you can't locate it locally any Chinese/spring greens will work well.

Cajun Shrimp Salad

- 200g/7oz large, raw & fresh king prawns/shrimps, peeled
- 75g/3oz pancetta/Italian bacon, cubed
- 1 tsp olive oil
- 2 tbsp freshly chopped flat leaf parsley
- ½ tsp each paprika, cayenne pepper, onion powder, garlic powder, oregano, sea salt & crushed chilli flakes
- 1 lemon
- 1 romaine lettuce, shredded
- ½ red onion, finely sliced
- 3 vine ripened tomatoes, sliced
- 3 tbsp balsamic vinegar
- 1 tbsp dijon mustard

- Cut the lemon in two. Squeeze the juice from one half and cut the other half into wedges.

- Combine together the fresh shrimp, lemon juice, paprika, cayenne pepper, onion powder, garlic powder, oregano, sea salt & crushed chillies and leave to marinate for a few minutes. Heat the olive oil in a frying pan and fry the shrimp on a high heat for 4-7 minutes or until they are pink and cooked through, add the parsley for the last minute or two of cooking.

- Meanwhile arrange the shredded lettuce, tomatoes and onion on a plate. Mix together the balsamic vinegar and dijon mustard to make a simple dressing and pour over the salad.

- When the prawns are ready arrange on the bed of salad and serve with lemon wedges on the side.

The cayenne pepper and crushed chilli flakes in this recipe pack quite a punch so feel free to alter the quantities to suit your own taste

Seafood 'Noodle' Soup

SERVES 1

- 250ml/1 cup chicken stock
- 2 garlic cloves, crushed
- 1 leek, finely chopped
- ½ tsp sea salt
- 1 tsp turmeric
- 2 tbsp freshly chopped flat leaf parsley
- 1 medium zucchini/courgette
- 75g/3oz raw, fresh, large prawns/shrimp
- 75g/3oz crab meat or boneless tilapia/cod fillet

180 calories

- Add the stock, garlic, leek, seafood, salt & turmeric to a pan and gently cook for 10-15 minutes until the seafood is cooked through.
- Meanwhile make your noodles by using a julienne/vegetable peeler to cut the zucchini/courgette into thin ribbons and then slice into 'noodle' size strips. When the soup is ready place the 'noodles' into the pan and gently warm through for a few minutes.
- Serve in a shallow bowl as a ramen style soup and sprinkle with parsley.

These zucchini noodles are a great alternative to traditional noodles.

Poached Wild Salmon & Tenderstem Broccoli

SERVES 1

- 150g/5oz boneless, skinless, wild salmon fillet
- 120ml/½ cup chicken stock
- 2 tbsp freshly chopped dill
- 150g/5oz tenderstem broccoli
- 2 tbsp lemon juice
- Sea salt & pepper to taste

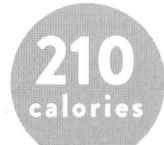

- Place the salmon and broccoli in a shallow pan with the stock and dill. Cover and leave to gently poach for aprox 10-12 minutes or until the vegetables are tender and the salmon is cooked through.

- Remove the broccoli and fish from the pan, discarding any remaining stock, and serve with lemon juice over the top.

Leave the tenderstem broccoli spears whole in this recipe and serve arranged around the salmon fillet.

Pan Fried Asparagus & Tilapia

SERVES 1

- 1 tbsp olive oil
- 150g/5oz boneless, skinless, fresh tilapia fillet
- 75g/3oz fresh asparagus spears
- 2 garlic cloves, crushed
- 1 red pepper, sliced
- 1 tbsp freshly chopped flat leaf parsley
- 1 tbsp lime juice
- ½ tsp paprika
- Sea salt & pepper to taste

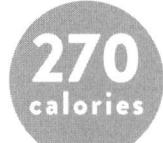

- Heat the oil and garlic in a frying pan and gently fry the sliced peppers and asparagus for a few minutes until tender.

- Remove to a plate and keep warm while you cook the tilapia.

- Increase the heat, season the fish and sprinkle with paprika. Fry on a high heat for a few minutes each side until the fish is cooked through.

- Remove from the pan, sprinkle with lime juice & parsley and serve with the warm asparagus and peppers.

Tilapia is a delicate white fish which is great with lime juice and paprika, however any firm white fish will work well in this dish.

Spiced Prawns & Cauliflower 'Rice'

SERVES 1

- 2 tsp olive oil
- 200g/7oz raw, fresh, king prawns/shrimps
- 2 garlic cloves, crushed
- 200g/7oz tinned chopped tomatoes
- 60ml/¼ cup coconut cream
- 1 onion, chopped
- 1 tbsp freshly chopped coriander
- 1 tsp each ground cumin, turmeric, cayenne pepper & coriander
- Cauliflower 'rice' (see page 77)
- Sea salt & pepper to taste

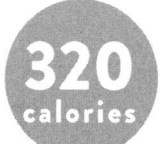
320 calories

- Gently fry the prawns, garlic and onion in the olive oil until the prawns begin to pink up.

- Add the ground spices and chopped tomatoes and continue to cook for 5-10 minutes until the prawns are cooked through and everything has combined well.

- Stir through the coconut cream and serve with cauliflower 'rice' sprinkled with fresh coriander.

You could bulk up this dish with some additional sliced peppers and chopped celery stalks if you have them to hand.

Japanese Tuna

SERVES 1

- 1 tsp olive oil
- 150g/5oz fresh, wild tuna steak
- 1 lime
- 1 tsp wasabi mustard
- 1 baby gem lettuce
- 2 vine ripened tomatoes, sliced
- 1 red onion, sliced
- Sea salt and pepper to taste

320 calories

- Mix together the wasabi and lime juice to make a paste.

- Arrange the lettuce, tomatoes and red onions in a shallow bowl.

- Put a frying pan on a high heat with the oil. Season the tuna steak and fry for 2-3 minutes each side.

- Remove from the pan, spread the wasabi mix over the top of the tuna and slice into diagonal strips. Arrange on top of the lettuce and serve.

Cooking the tuna for 2 mins each side will leave it rare - the best way to enjoy fresh tuna steak. However feel free to increase cooking time if you prefer.

Italian Bacon Mussels

SERVES 1

- 1 tsp olive oil
- A dozen raw, fresh, cleaned mussels
- 50g/2oz pancetta/Italian bacon, cubed
- 2 garlic cloves, crushed
- 250g/1 cup fish stock
- Juice of 1 lemon
- 3 tbsp freshly chopped flat leaf parsley
- Sea salt & pepper to taste

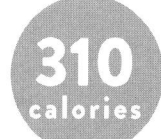

- Place the bacon, garlic & oil in a large saucepan and fry for a few minutes.
- Add the mussels and stock, increase the heat to high and leave to cook for 5-8 minutes or until the mussels open and the stock reduces.
- Tip the contents of the pan into a large bowl (discarding any mussels which are not fully open).
- Sprinkle with parsley, squeeze the lemon juice over the top and serve.

Use the freshest mussels available and serve with bread to mop up all the delicious bacon & stock juices.

Tandoori Prawn Skewers

SERVES 1

- 1 tsp olive oil
- 200g/7oz large, fresh, raw prawns/shrimps
- 1 tsp each ground cumin, turmeric, coriander & chilli powder
- ½ tsp each ground ginger & garam masala
- 1 tbsp lemon juice
- 2 garlic cloves, crushed
- 1 baby gem lettuce, shredded
- 1 large pepper, cut into pieces
- 1 onion, cut into pieces
- ½ lemon cut into wedges
- 3 large metal skewers
- Sea salt & pepper to taste

250 calories

- Mix together the olive oil, lemon juice, ground spices & garlic to form a paste (add a little water if needed).

- Season the prawns/shrimps, onion & pepper pieces, and smother in the spice paste. Place in a dish and leave for up to 1 hour to marinate.

- Skewer the prawns/shrimps, pepper & onion pieces in turn to make two or three kebabs. Grill under a medium/high heat for 5-7 minutes each side, or until the prawns/shrimps are cooked through and the vegetable pieces are tender (take care handling the skewers as they will get hot).

- Plate up the skewers along with the shredded lettuce and serve with the lemon wedges.

Any type of large raw prawn/shrimp is good for this dish, use peeled or unpeeled depending on your own preference.

Mediterranean Fish Stew

SERVES 1

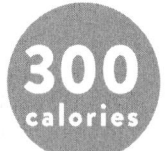

- 1 tbsp olive oil
- 75g/3oz small peeled fresh prawns/shrimps
- 75g/3oz boneless, fresh, meaty white fish fillet, cut into chunks
- 1 onion, chopped
- 2 garlic cloves, crushed
- 60ml/¼ cup fish stock
- 125g/4oz fresh tomatoes, finely chopped
- Splash dry white wine
- 1 tbsp sundried tomato paste
- 1 tbsp each freshly chopped rosemary & basil
- 1 bay leaf
- Salt & pepper to taste

- Gently sauté the onion, sundried tomato paste & garlic in a little olive oil for a few minutes.

- Add all the other ingredients to the pan. Cover and leave to cook for 15-20 minutes or until everything is cooked through.

- Adjust the seasoning, remove the bay leaf and serve.

Feel free to use tinned tomatoes if you don't have fresh tomatoes to hand.

Stuffed Lemon Sole

SERVES 1

- 1 tsp olive oil
- 150g/5oz skinless, fresh, boneless lemon sole
- 1 garlic clove, crushed
- ½ onion, chopped
- 1 tbsp freshly chopped flat leaf parsley
- 50g/2oz chestnut mushrooms, chopped
- 3 vine ripened tomatoes, halved
- 50g/2oz rocket leaves
- ½ lemon cut into wedges
- Salt & pepper to taste

240 calories

- Slice the lemon sole fillet to create a cavity for stuffing.

- Gently sauté the mushrooms, garlic & onions in the olive oil for a few minutes and stuff into the fillet.

- Place the fish along with the tomatoes on a grill pan. Season well, brush with a little olive oil and grill for 8-12 minutes or until the fish is properly cooked through and the tomatoes are tender.

- Serve with the rocket salad and lemon wedges.

Lemon sole has a delicate flavour which is gently complemented with the ingredients in this dish.

Sweet Wild Salmon & Asparagus

SERVES 1

- 150g/5oz thick skinless, boneless wild salmon fillet
- 1 tsp runny honey
- ½ tsp olive oil
- ½ lemon cut into wedges
- 100g/3 ½oz asparagus spears
- Sea salt & pepper to taste

280 calories

- Mix together the honey and oil and brush on the salmon and asparagus.
- Place under the grill on a medium/high heat. Season well and cook for 10-12 minutes or until the salmon is properly cooked through and the asparagus are tender.
- Serve with lemon wedges on the side.

Use a thick piece of salmon for this recipe. You could add a pinch of crushed chillies to the asparagus spears for an extra 'kick' too.

Homemade Fish Goujons

SERVES 1

- 150g/5oz skinless, boneless, fresh cod or haddock fillets
- 1 tbsp olive oil
- 2 free range eggs
- 4 tbsp bread crumbs
- 2 tsp each garlic & onion powder
- ½ lemon
- 2 tsp dried basil
- Sea salt & pepper to taste

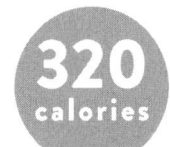

- First slice the fish fillets into strips and season well.

- Combine the bread crumbs, garlic and onion powder on a plate and beat the eggs in a bowl.

- Cover each fish strip with bread crumbs by rolling them on the plate and then dip each strip in the egg.

- Heat the oil in a frying pan and fry the fish strips in the sizzling oil for a few minutes until cooked through.

- Serve with the lemon wedges.

Ensure your goujons are nicely browned by increasing the heat and the oil quantity a little if needed.

The Rapid 800

vegetable
dishes & sides

Aromatic Cilantro Mushrooms

SERVES 1

- 1 tbsp olive oil
- 150g/5oz chestnut mushrooms, sliced
- 1 garlic clove, crushed
- 1 tsp each cumin & caraway seeds
- ½ tsp each ground cumin and nutmeg
- 2 tbsp freshly chopped cilantro (coriander)
- 2 tbsp lemon juice
- Sea salt & pepper to taste

- Heat the oil in a pan and gently begin frying the cumin and caraway seeds.
- Add the mushrooms and garlic and cook for a minute or two.
- Add the ground cumin, nutmeg & lemon juice and cook until the mushrooms are tender.
- Season, sprinkle with chopped coriander and serve.

This is a lovely side dish, which can be served with fish or meat. Alternatively bulk up with a salad and serve as a main course.

Basil & Vegetable Bake

SERVES 1

- 1 tbsp olive oil
- 2 garlic cloves, crushed
- 2 tbsp balsamic vinegar
- 1 red onion, sliced
- ½ zucchini/courgette
- ½ eggplant/aubergine
- ½ tsp sea salt
- 60ml/¼ cup tomato pasatta/sieved tomatoes
- 3 tbsp freshly chopped basil
- Sea salt & pepper to taste

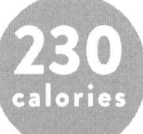
230 calories

- Preheat the oven to 180°C/350F/Gas Mark 5.

- Use a vegetable peeler/julienne to cut the zucchini/courgette into ribbons. Slice the eggplant/aubergine thinly and sprinkle salt over them both. Mix well and leave to draw out the moisture for 10 minutes.

- Rinse with water and sauté in a frying pan with the olive oil.

- Add the onion, garlic & balsamic vinegar and cook until the vegetables are tender.

- Add the sieved tomatoes, mix and place in an ovenproof dish. Bake for 20-30 minutes until piping hot.

- Sprinkle with fresh basil and serve.

You could also use rosemary and/or tarragon in this vegetable bake to complement the dish.

Spiced Roasted Squash

SERVES 1

- ½ butternut squash, peeled and cut into small cubes
- 1 tbsp olive oil
- 1 garlic clove, crushed
- ½ tsp each garam masala, turmeric, sea salt, cumin, paprika & coriander

180 calories

- Preheat the oven to 180C/350F/Gas Mark 5.
- Combine all the ingredients in a bowl. Make sure the squash is completely coated with the oil, garlic and spices.
- Transfer to a baking tray and cook for 20-30 minutes or until the squash is tender and begins to brown.

You could try adding a little honey to this dish along with the spices to caramelize the squash for an even sweeter taste.

Cauliflower 'Rice'

SERVES 1

- ¼ head large cauliflower
- Sea salt & pepper to taste

- Place the cauliflower in a food processor and whizz into breadcrumb-size pieces.
- Season, put in a dish, cover and microwave for 2-3 minutes until tender.

Zucchini 'Noodles'

SERVES 1

- 1 medium zucchini/courgette
- Sea salt & pepper to taste

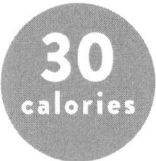

- Make the noodles by using a julienne/vegetable peeler to cut the zucchini/courgette into thin ribbons and then slice into 'noodle' size strips.
- Season, put in a dish, cover and microwave for 2-3 minutes until tender.

HIIT **Plan Workouts**

High Intensity Interval Training is a super fast and really effective way to workout. The short but intense bursts of exercise with rest in between makes your heart work harder and so increases cardio strength, improves metabolism and as a result helps your body burn more calories both during and after your workout. HiiT can also help control blood sugar levels.

It's a very efficient way to train to build a leaner, fitter body and because no equipment is required you can workout at home or just about anywhere.

We have compiled **3** core workouts to perform throughout each week. Choose one workout to perform per day and use the remaining 4 days to rest. Try to alternate between training and rest days. Each workout lasts for approximately 15 mins and a simple explanation of how to correctly perform each exercise in the set is explained in the following pages.

It's very important to warm up your muscles and joints before beginning any exercise to prevent injury and to make sure you perform each repetition to the best of your ability. Stretch for at least 2 minutes before your workout (see page 94 for stretches), then warm up by jogging on the spot for two minutes.

Always cool down and stretch again at the end of your workout. See workouts on p94.

Tips

- Warm up and cool down before and after each workout
- Have a bottle of water to drink from between sets
- Remember to breathe through each exercise
- Keep your core tight & give maximum effort
- Focus on maintaining correct posture & form for each exercise

HIIT **Workout One**

- Exercise 1: **HIGH KNEES** 20 secs | 10 secs rest
- Exercise 2: **BODYWEIGHT SQUATS** 20 secs | 10 secs rest
- Exercise 3: **JUMPING JACKS** 20 secs | 10 secs rest
- Exercise 4: **SIDE LUNGE** 20 secs | 10 secs rest
- Exercise 5: **TRICEP DIPS** 20 secs | 10 secs rest
- Exercise 6: **MOUNTAIN CLIMBERS** 20 secs | 10 sec rest
- Exercise 7: **BUTT KICKS** 20 secs | 2 minute rest

Repeat for 2 more sets

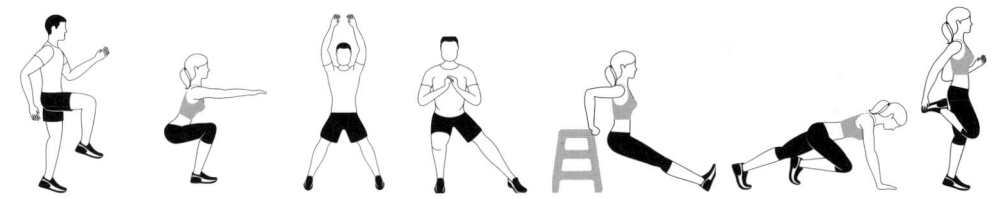

Perform each exercise as many times as possible within 20 seconds. Rest for 10 seconds then perform the next exercise again for 20 secs with a 10 sec rest in between exercises. Repeat until all 7 exercises have been completed.

Rest for 2 minutes then repeat the whole set two more times with a 2 minute rest in between.

Remember that these are high intensity workouts so try to push yourself to get as many repetitions of each exercise with the correct form within the 20 second period.

High Knees

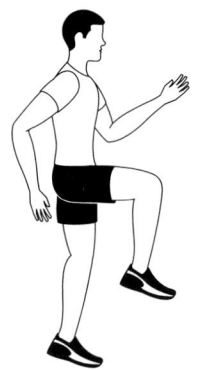 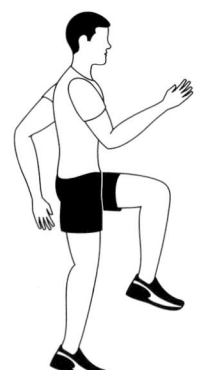

Stand straight with the feet hip width apart, looking straight ahead and arms hanging down by your side. Jump from one foot to the other at the same time lifting your knees as high as possible, hip height is advisable. The arms should be following the motion. Try holding your hands just above the hips so that your knees touch the palms of your hands as you lift your knees.

Bodyweight Squats

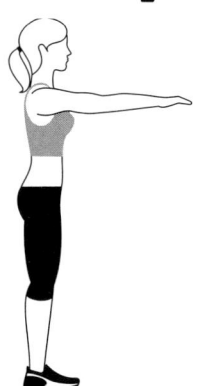 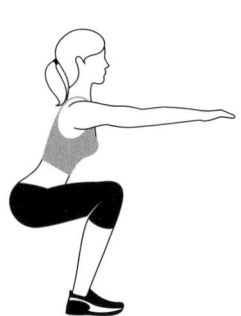

Stand with your feet shoulder width apart with your arms extended in front of you. Begin the movement by flexing your knees and hips, sitting back with your hips until your thighs are parallel with the floor in the full squat position. Quickly reverse the motion until you return to the starting position as you keep your head and chest up.

Jumping Jacks

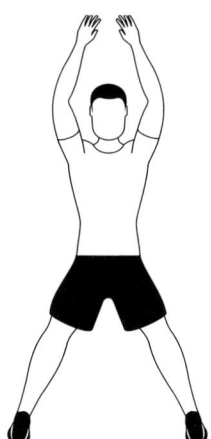

Stand with your feet together and your hands down by your side. In one motion jump your feet out to the side and raise your arms above your head. Immediately reverse by jumping back to the starting position.

Side Lunge

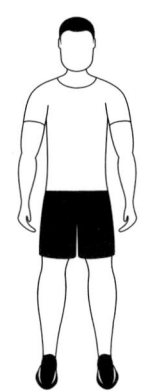

Stand with your knees and hips slightly bent, feet shoulder-width apart and the head and chest up. Keeping your left leg straight, step out to the side with your right leg and bend at your right knee transferring weight to your right side. Extend through the right leg to return to the starting position. Repeat on the left leg.

Tricep Dips

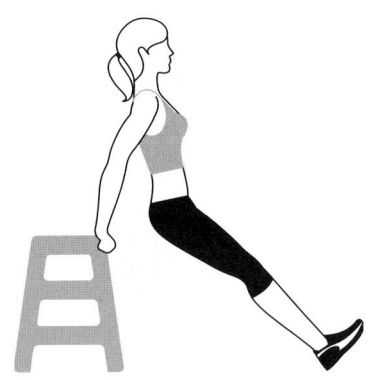 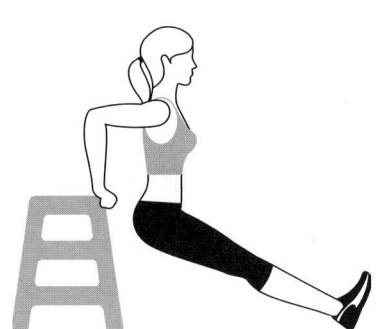

Position your hands shoulder-width apart on a secure bench or stable chair. Slide off the front of the bench with your legs extended out in front of you. Straighten your arms, keeping a slight bend in your elbows. Slowly bend your elbows to lower your body toward the floor until your elbows are at about a 90-degree angle. At this point press down into the bench or chair to straighten your elbows, returning to the starting position.

Mountain Climber

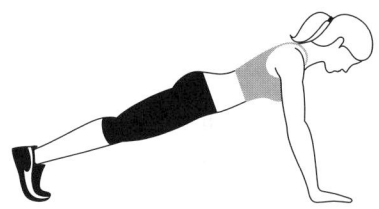 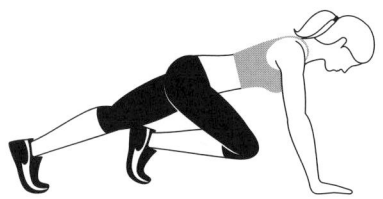

Begin in a pushup position, with your weight supported by your hands and toes. Flexing the knee and hip, bring one leg towards the corresponding arm. Explosively reverse the positions of your legs, extending the bent leg until the leg is straight and supported by the toe, and bringing the other foot up with the hip and knee flexed. Repeat in an alternating fashion.

Butt Kicks

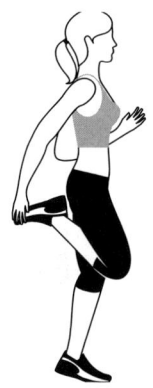 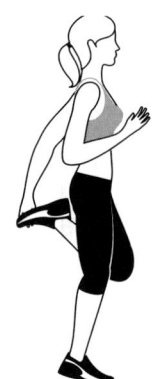

Stand with your legs shoulder-width apart and your arms bent. Flex the right knee and kick your right heel up toward your glutes. Bring the right foot back down while flexing your left knee and kicking your left foot up toward your glutes. Repeat in a continuous movement.

TOP TIP

Warm up properly. By warming up your muscles you will reduce the chances of injury or strain. Warm up with jogging on the spot, gentle jumping jacks and stretches (see page 94) for at least 2 minutes.

HIIT Workout Two

- Exercise 1: **BURPEES** 20 secs | 10 secs rest
- Exercise 2: **JAB SQUATS** 20 secs | 10 secs rest
- Exercise 3: **MUMMY KICKS** 20 secs | 10 secs rest
- Exercise 4: **SIDE SKATER** 20 secs | 10 secs rest
- Exercise 5: **TUCK JUMP** 20 secs | 10 secs rest
- Exercise 6: **SPRINTS** 20 secs | 10 sec rest
- Exercise 7: **HEISMAN** 20 secs | 2 minute rest

Repeat for 2 more sets

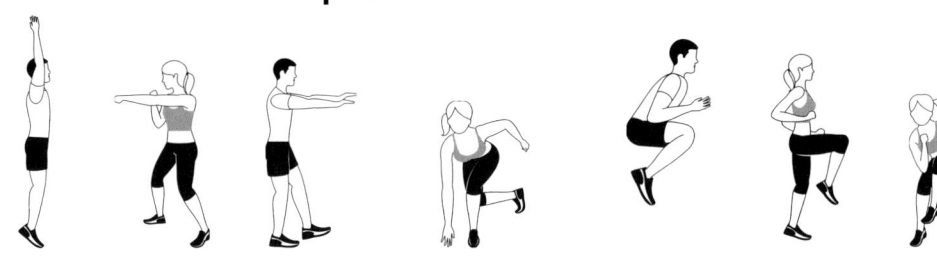

Perform each exercise as many times as possible within 20 seconds. Rest for 10 seconds then perform the next exercise again for 20 secs with a 10 sec rest in between exercises. Repeat until all 7 exercises have been completed.

Rest for 2 minutes then repeat the whole set two more times with a 2 minute rest in between.

Remember that these are high intensity workouts so try to push yourself to get as many repetitions of each exercise with the correct form within the 20 second period.

Burpees

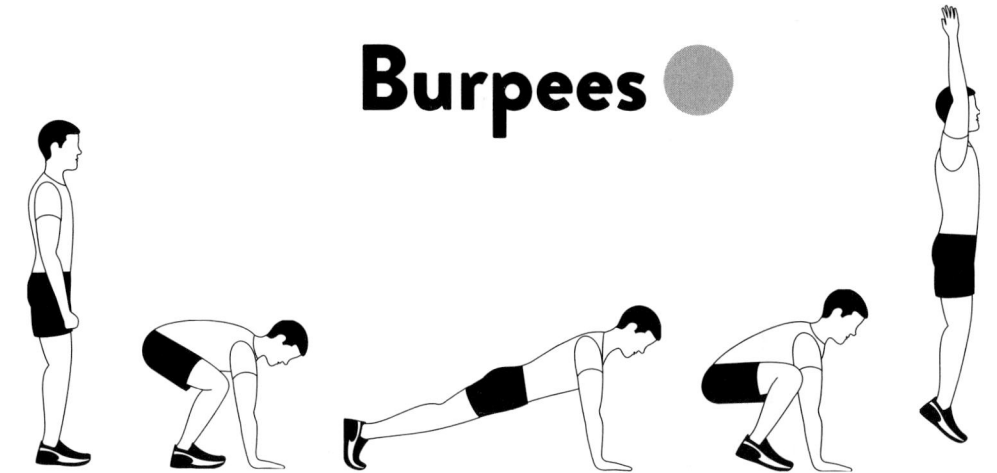

Stand with your feet shoulder-width apart, with your arms at your sides. Push your hips back, bend your knees, and lower your body into a squat before placing your hands on the floor directly in front of, and just inside, your feet. Jump your feet back to land in a plank position forming a straight line from head to toe with a straight back. Jump your feet back again so that they land just outside of your hands. Reach your arms over head and explosively jump up into the air. Land and immediately lower back into a squat for your next repetition.

Jab Squats

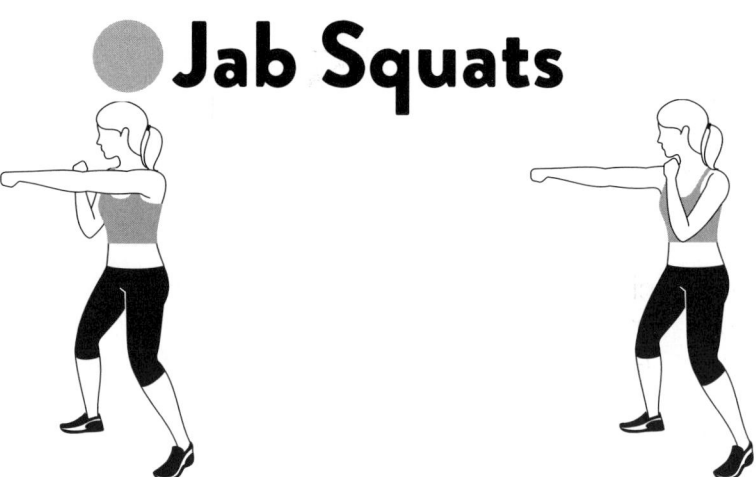

Start in a half squat position with your feet shoulder-width apart and knees slightly bent. Bring your arms up so the palms are facing the sides of your face. Clench your fists. Use sharp movements to lengthen your right arm in front in a punching motion then return to the starting position immediately punching out your left arm. Keep switching sides in a quick powerful motion.

Mummy Kicks

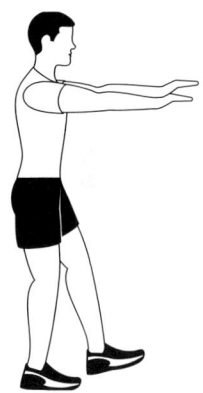 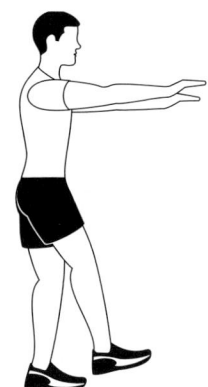

Begin by standing with your arms extended straight out in front. Perform light hop kicks with your feet while simultaneously criss-crossing your hands. Alternate the motion of your arms and hands as you swap between legs. Keep your core tight.

Side Skater

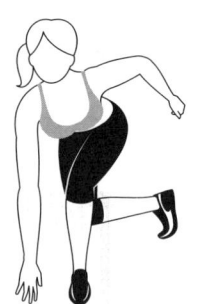 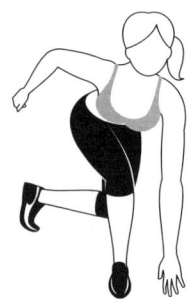

Start in a squat position with your left leg bent at the knee and your right arm parallel for balance. Your right leg is extended but still bent at the knee behind you. Jump sideways to the right, landing on your right leg. Bring your left leg behind you with your left arm extended and fingers touching the floor. Keep your back straight and your core engaged. Reverse direction by jumping to the left.

Tuck Jump

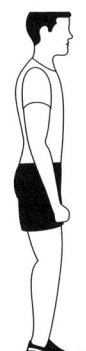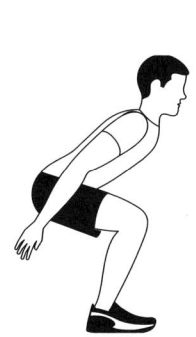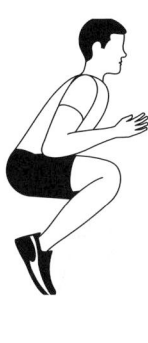

Begin in a standing position with knees slightly bent and arms at your sides. Bend your knees and lower your body quickly into a squat position, then explosively jump upwards bringing your knees up towards your chest.

Sprints

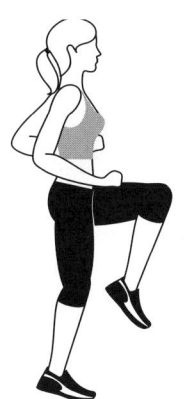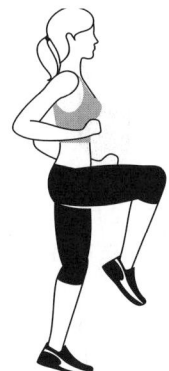

Standing with your feet shoulder-width apart, move your arms and torso as though you are running as fast as you can on the spot. Move feet and legs as little as possible avoiding twisting from side to side.

Heisman

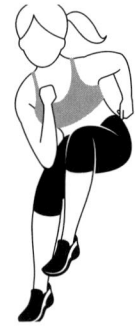 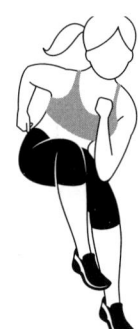

Begin by standing with feet shoulder-width apart and knees slightly bent. Jump onto your right foot while pulling your left knee up and towards the left shoulder. Next jump onto your left foot while pulling your right knee towards the right shoulder. Continue the movement in a quick motion, switching between legs.

TOP TIP

Use a timer or stopwatch to precisely time each exercise and your rest time. There are many free apps available online. Try searching for 'tabata timer app'.

HIIT Workout Three

- Exercise 1: **SIT UPS** 20 secs | 10 secs rest
- Exercise 2: **BICYCLE CRUNCH** 20 secs | 10 secs rest
- Exercise 3: **MUMMY KICKS** 20 secs | 10 secs rest
- Exercise 4: **JAB SQUATS** 20 secs | 10 secs rest
- Exercise 5: **LATERALS** 20 secs | 10 secs rest
- Exercise 6: **MOUNTAIN CLIMBER** 20 secs | 10 sec rest
- Exercise 7: **TAP UPS** 20 secs | 2 minute rest

Repeat for 2 more sets

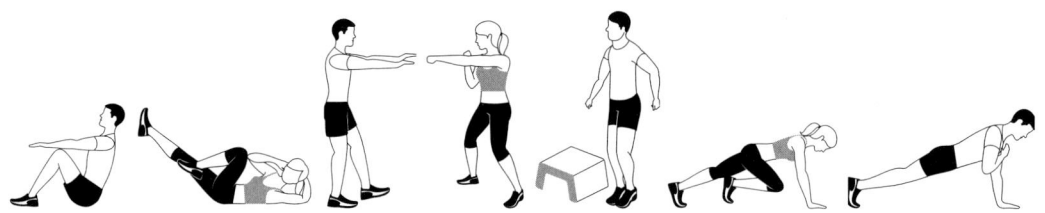

Perform each exercise as many times as possible within 20 seconds. Rest for 10 seconds then perform the next exercise again for 20 secs with a 10 sec rest in between exercises. Repeat until all 7 exercises have been completed.

Rest for 2 minutes then repeat the whole set two more times with a 2 minute rest in between.

Remember that these are high intensity workouts so try to push yourself to get as many repetitions of each exercise with the correct form within the 20 second period.

Sit Ups

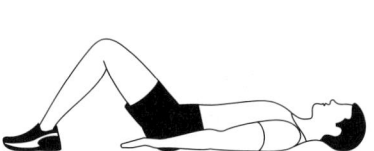 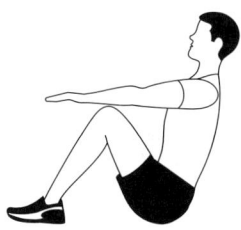

Lie on your back with your knees bent and your arms extended at your sides. and your feet flat on the floor. Engage your core and slowly curl your upper back off the floor towards your knees with your arms extended out. Roll back down to the starting position.

Bicycle Crunch

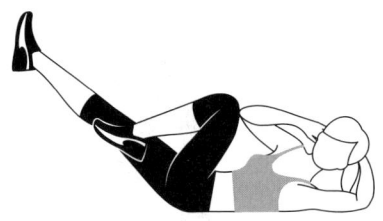 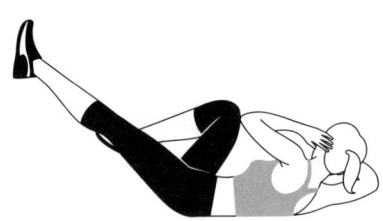

Lie face up and place your hands at the side of your head (do not pull on the back of your head). Make sure your core is tight and the small of your back is pushed hard against the floor. Lift your knees in toward your chest while lifting your shoulder blades off the floor. Rotate to the right, bringing the left elbow towards the right knee as you extend the other leg into the air. Switch sides, bringing the right elbow towards the left knee. Alternate each side in a pedaling motion..

Mummy Kicks

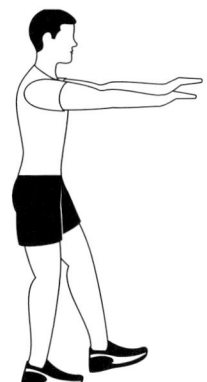 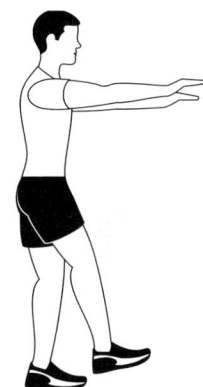

Begin by standing with your arms extended straight out in front. Perform light hop kicks with your feet while simultaneously criss-crossing your hands. Alternate the motion of your arms and hands as you swap between legs. Keep your core tight.

Jab Squats

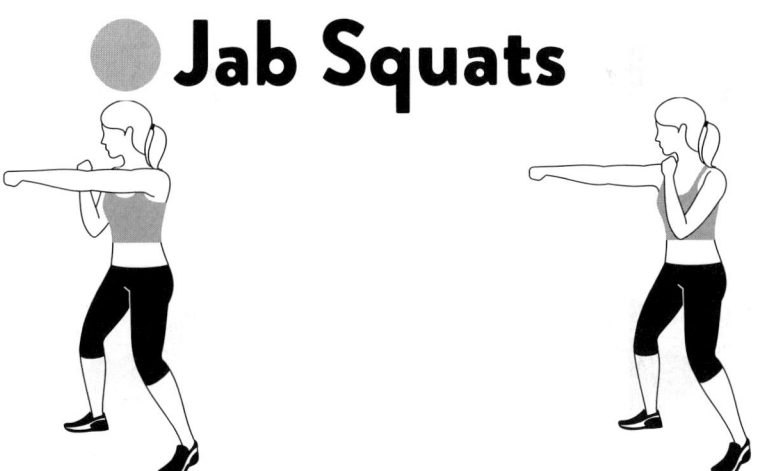

Start in a half squat position with your feet shoulder-width apart and knees slightly bent. Bring your arms up so the palms are facing the sides of your face. Clench your fists. Use sharp movements to lengthen your right arm in front in a punching motion then return to the starting position immediately punching out your left arm. Keep switching sides in a quick powerful motion.

Laterals

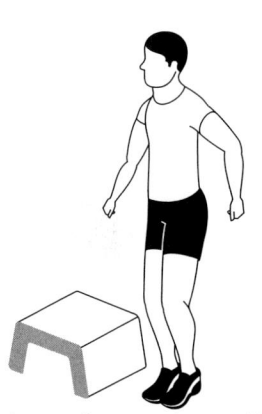 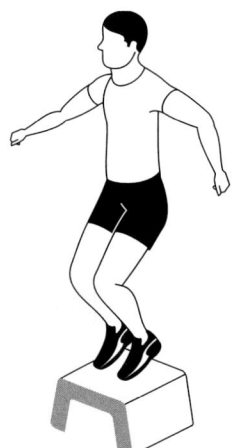

Stand beside a step or box. Position into a quarter squat then jump up and over to the right landing on the box with both feet landing together. Bring your knees high enough to ensure your feet clear the box. Jump over to the other side and repeat, this time jumping to the left.

Mountain Climber

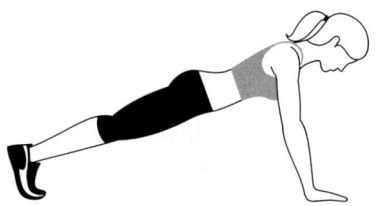 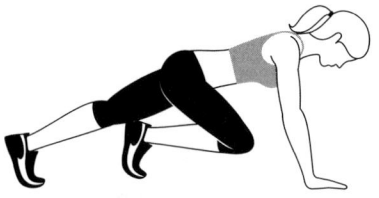

Begin in a pushup position, with your weight supported by your hands and toes. Flexing the knee and hip, bring one leg towards the corresponding arm. Explosively reverse the positions of your legs, extending the bent leg until the leg is straight and supported by the toe, and bringing the other foot up with the hip and knee flexed. Repeat in an alternating fashion.

Tap Ups

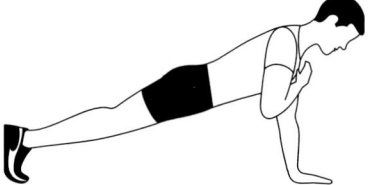

Begin in a pushup/plank position with your hands slightly wider than shoulder-width apart. Bend your elbows to lower your body to the floor just like a normal pushup. Pause, press back up to the starting position then tap one shoulder with the opposite side's hand. Repeat tapping the opposite shoulder.

TOP TIP

Work as hard as you can in each 30 sec burst. This is high intensity training so give maximum effort while maintaining correct form for each exercise.

Straight Leg Calf Stretch

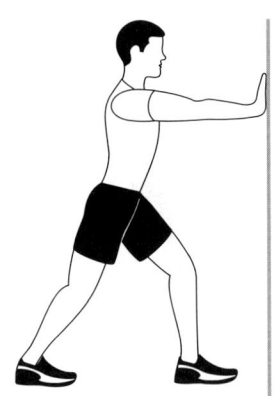 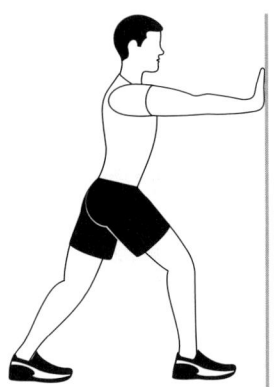

Place both hands on a wall with arms extended. Lean against the wall with right leg bent forward and left leg extended behind with knee straight and feet positioned directly forward. Push rear heal to floor and move hips slightly forward holding the stretch for 10 secs. Repeat with opposite leg.

Shoulder Stretch

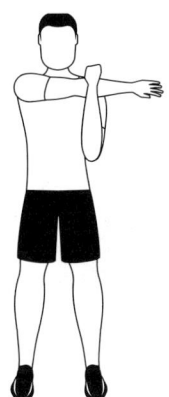 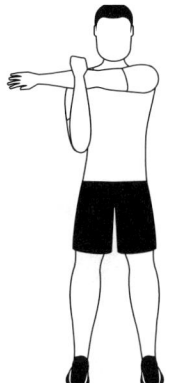

The right arm is placed over the left shoulder. Position the wrist on your left arm to the elbow of your right arm gently pushing towards the shoulder. Swap shoulders.

STRETCHES

Standing Quadricep Stretch

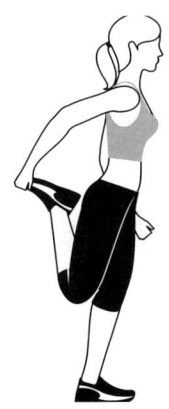 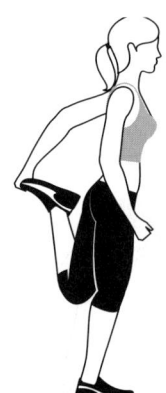

Begin by standing with your feet hip-width apart. Bend your right leg backwards grasping the right foot to bring your heel toward your buttocks. Hold for 5-10 secs then repeat for left leg. Use your opposite arm to balance if need be.

Lower Back Stretch

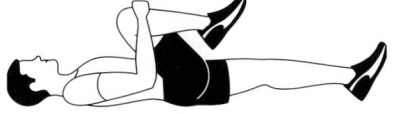 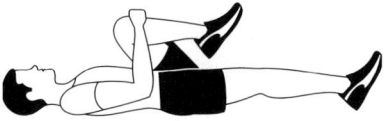

Begin by lying flat on your back with toes pointed upward. Slowly bend your right knee and pull your leg up to you chest, wrapping your arms around your thigh and hands clasped around the knee or shin. Gently pull the knee towards your chest and hold for 10 secs. Repeat on left leg.

STRETCHES

Cat Cow Stretch

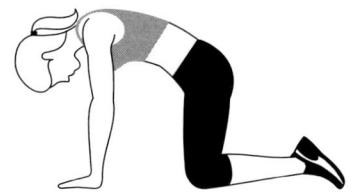
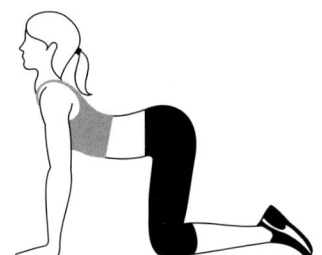

Begin with your hands and knees on the floor. Exhale while rounding your spine up towards the ceiling, pulling your belly button up towards your spine, and engaging your core. Inhale while arching your back and letting your tummy relax.